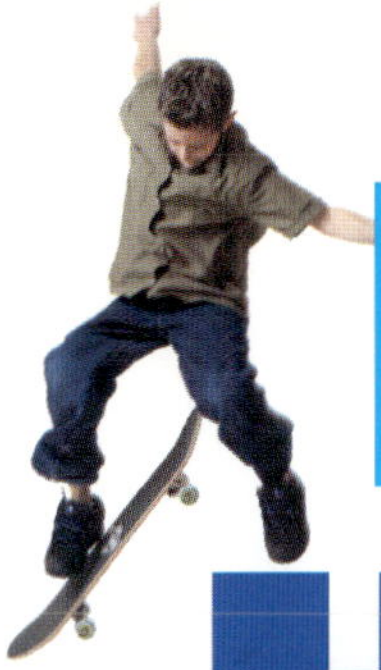

Having Healthful Habits

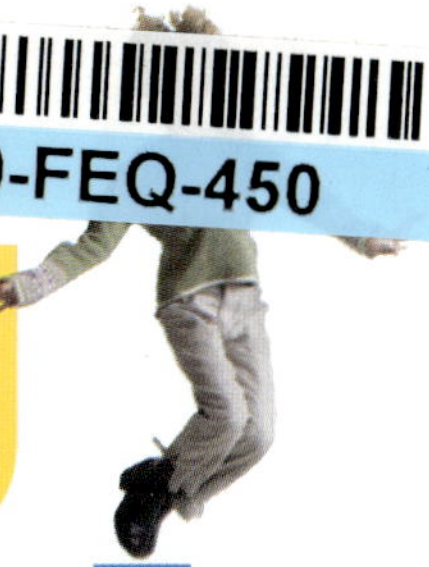

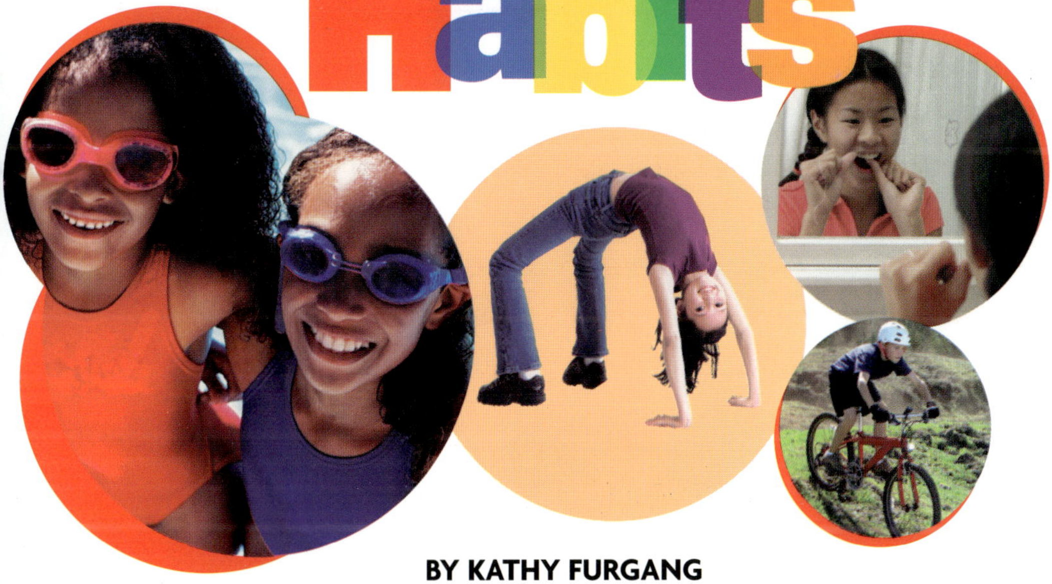

BY KATHY FURGANG

Table of Contents

Introduction 2
Chapter 1 Food for Life 6
Chapter 2 Fitness for Life 12
Chapter 3 A Healthy Look 18
Chapter 4 Preventing Illness.................. 21
Chapter 5 Safety and First Aid 24
Glossary 31
Index 32

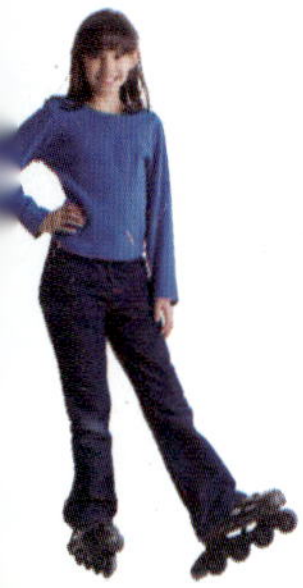

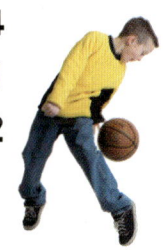

Introduction

When you think about what it means to be healthy, do you think of visiting a doctor, exercising, or eating the right foods? Good! These are important ways to stay healthy.

There are many other things you can do to be healthy as well. Having good relationships with friends and family helps your mind stay sharp and healthy. Talking about your emotions helps you have a healthy mind. Eating well, getting rest, and being relaxed help you have a healthy body.

Social health, mental health, and physical health are all part of **wellness**. When you have a healthy body and mind, you can do your best and feel your best.

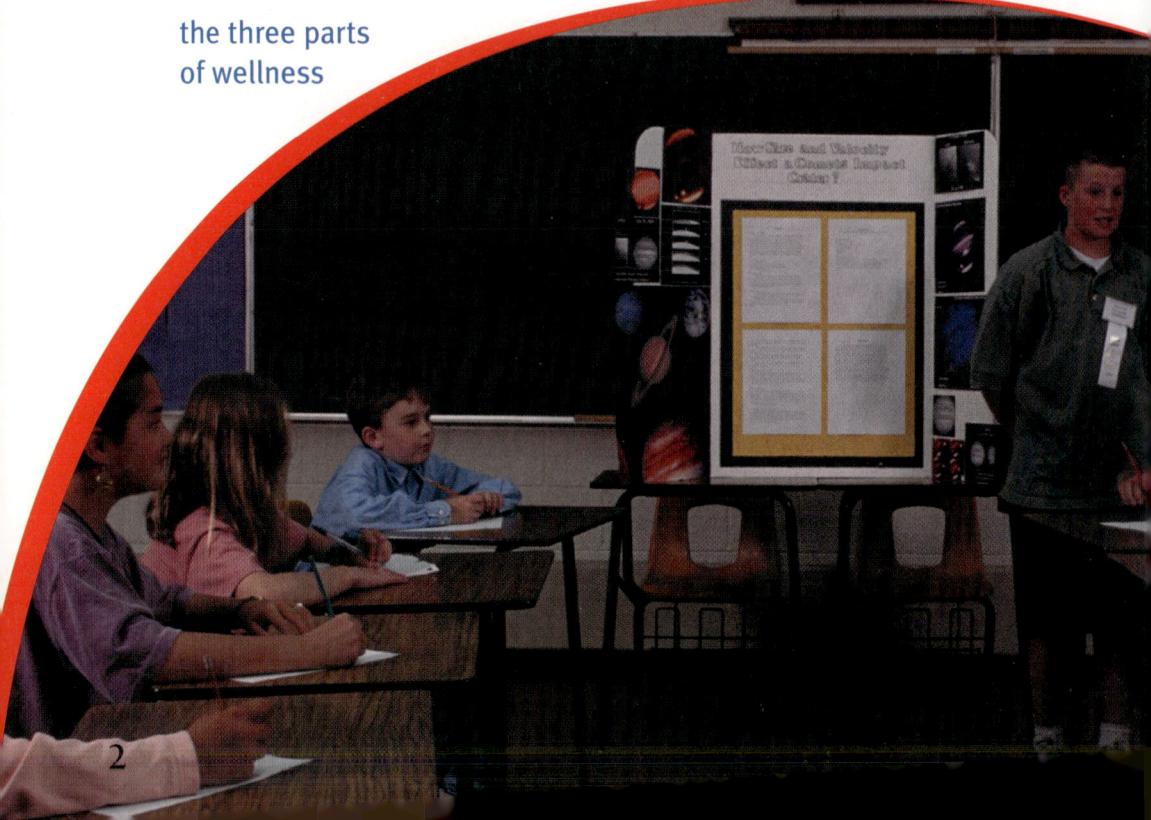

the three parts of wellness

How you get along with people is an important factor in your social health. Friends, family, teachers, and anyone you come in contact with can affect your social health. Social health involves your experiences with others.

Mental health involves your emotions and feelings. Expressing your feelings and dealing with stress in healthful ways help you improve your mental health.

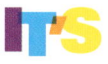

Stress is one of your body's reactions to the world around you. Your heart races, your muscles become tense, and you may feel nervous. Too much stress over time can make you more likely to get colds and other illnesses.

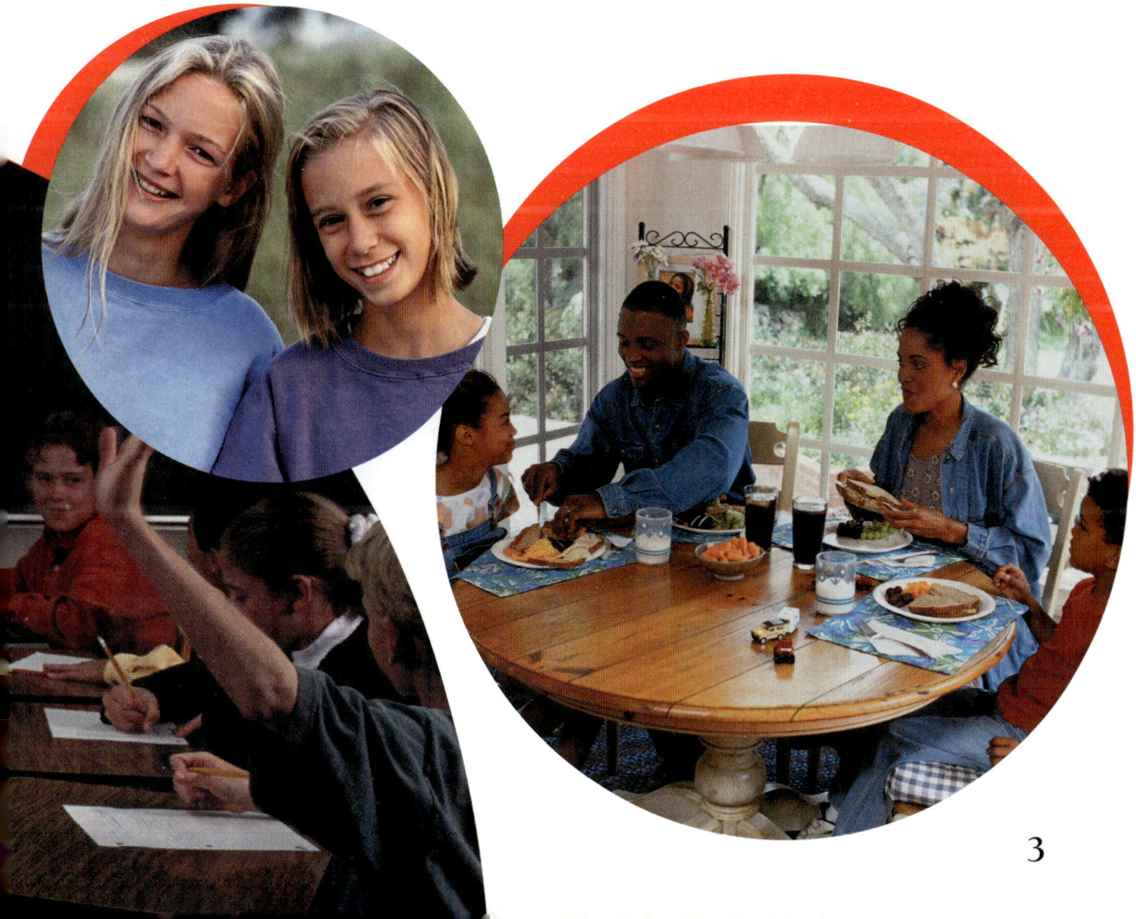

Physical health involves having your body in the best possible condition so it can do whatever you ask it to do. There are five major areas of physical health—nutrition, fitness, grooming, illness prevention, and personal safety. In this book, you will learn about each area and explore ways to develop good habits for a healthy body. If you develop healthful habits now, they can last you a lifetime. Healthful habits can even help you live longer.

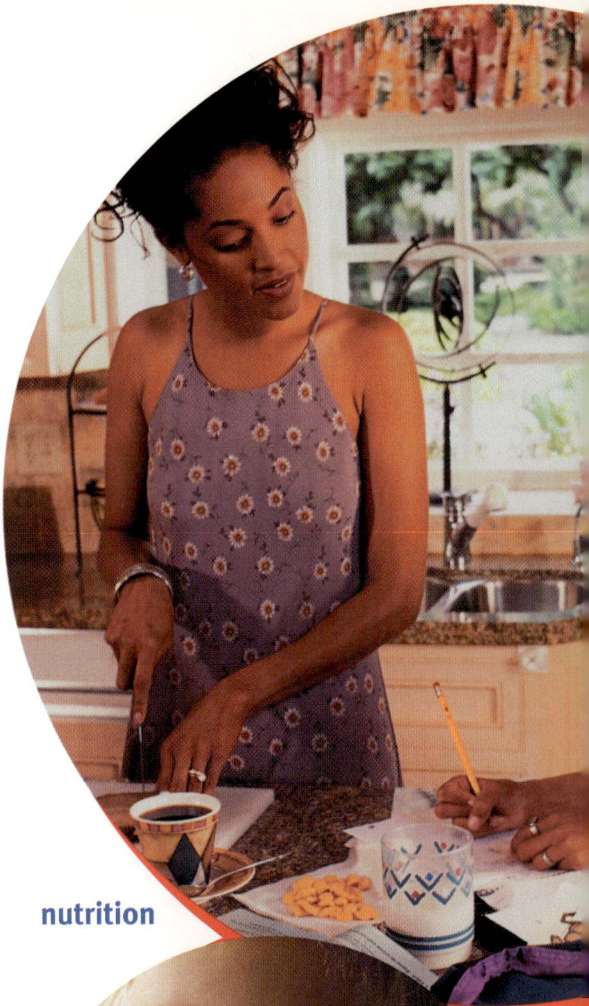

nutrition

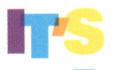

In 1900, the average life span for Americans was about 47 years. The average life span for Americans today is close to 80 years, due to improvements in healthcare and medicine. The longest anyone has ever lived is 122 years.

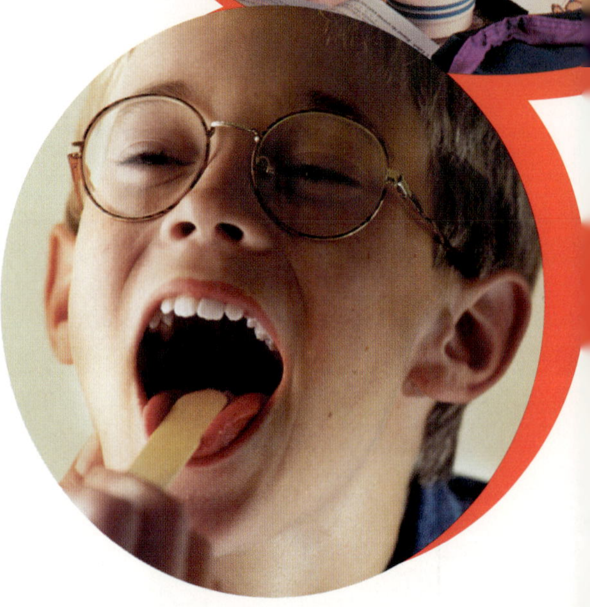

illness prevention

INTRODUCTION

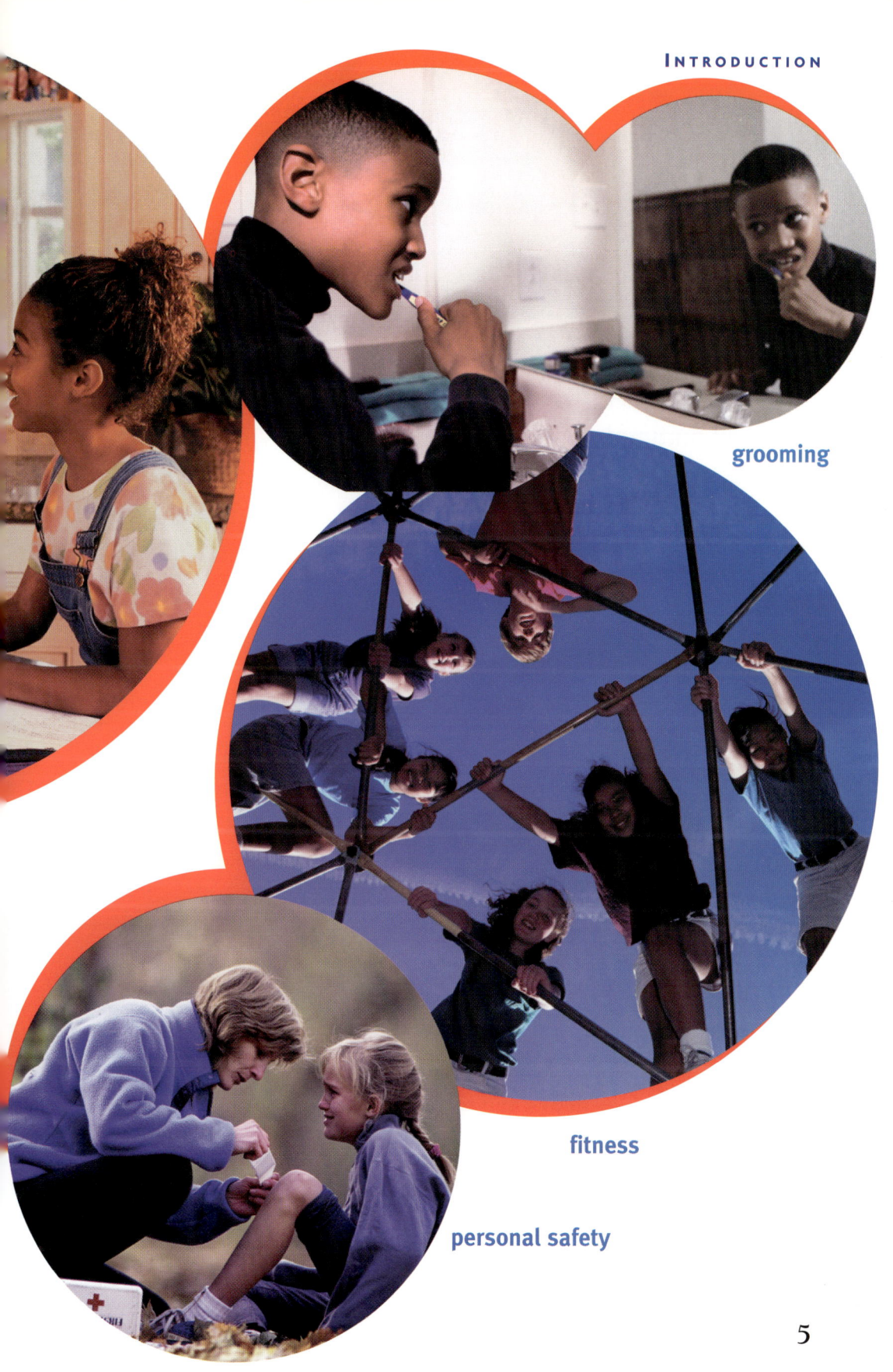

grooming

fitness

personal safety

5

CHAPTER 1

Food for Life

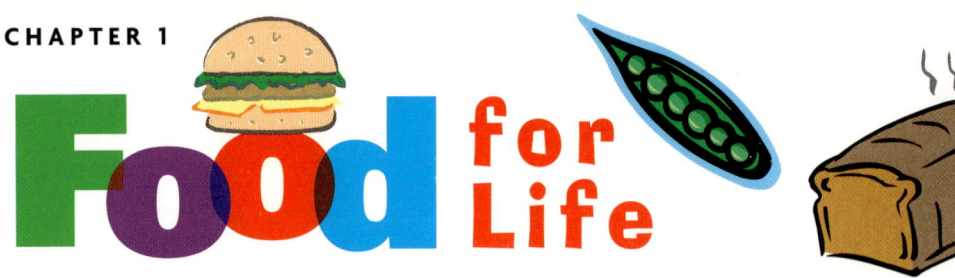

Food is one of the most important parts of good health. You need food to live! Your body needs **nutrients** that are found only in foods. Your body uses some of these nutrients as sources of energy throughout the day.

Nutrients also help your body grow, your brain function, and your cells repair themselves. Different nutrients help the body in different ways. The chart shows six main types of nutrients and how your body uses them.

Nutrients Checklist

Nutrient	What it does	Where to find it
Carbohydrates	supply body with much of its energy	bread, rice, potatoes, cereals, noodles, fruits, vegetables
Proteins	supply energy; help cells grow and repair themselves	eggs, cheese, milk, fish, meats, beans, nuts
Vitamins	help regulate body functions and fight disease; help with new cell growth	fruits, vegetables, milk, meats, breads, eggs
Minerals	help regulate body functions; build new cells; form bones and teeth	fruits, vegetables, milk, meats, breads, eggs
Fats	supply energy; help store some vitamins	plant oils, butter, milk, ice cream, meats
Water	helps with digestion, removing waste products, and regulating body temperature	drinking water, milk, soups, juices, fruits, vegetables

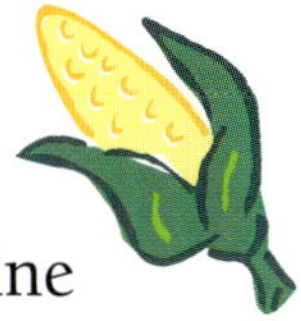

How can you determine what nutrients are in the foods you eat and drink each day?

Try this activity.
What you need
- paper
- pen or pencil

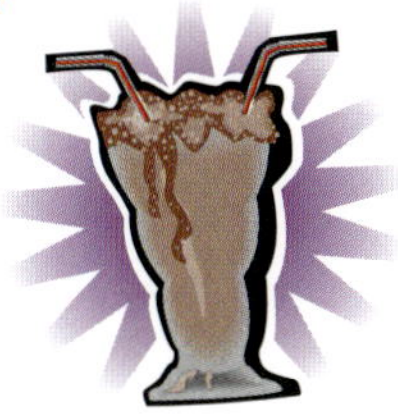

What to do
1. Write down everything you eat for one day. Be sure to include snacks and drinks.
2. Compare your list to the nutrients checklist on the opposite page. What nutrients are in each food you ate?
3. Make a chart of the information. Write the nutrients in one column and the food in the other. Divide foods such as sandwiches into several categories if necessary.

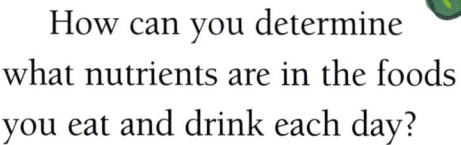

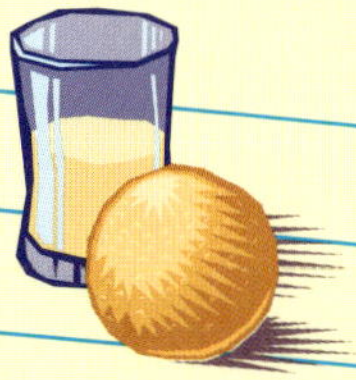

carbohydrates	cereal, bread
proteins	turkey
vitamins	milk
minerals	carrot sticks
fats	mayonnaise
	potato chips
water	drinking water
	orange juice

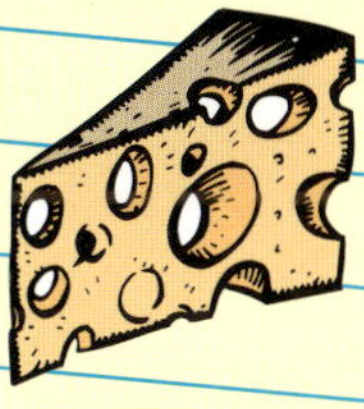

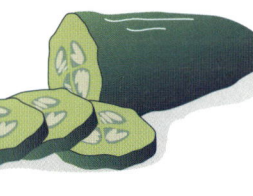

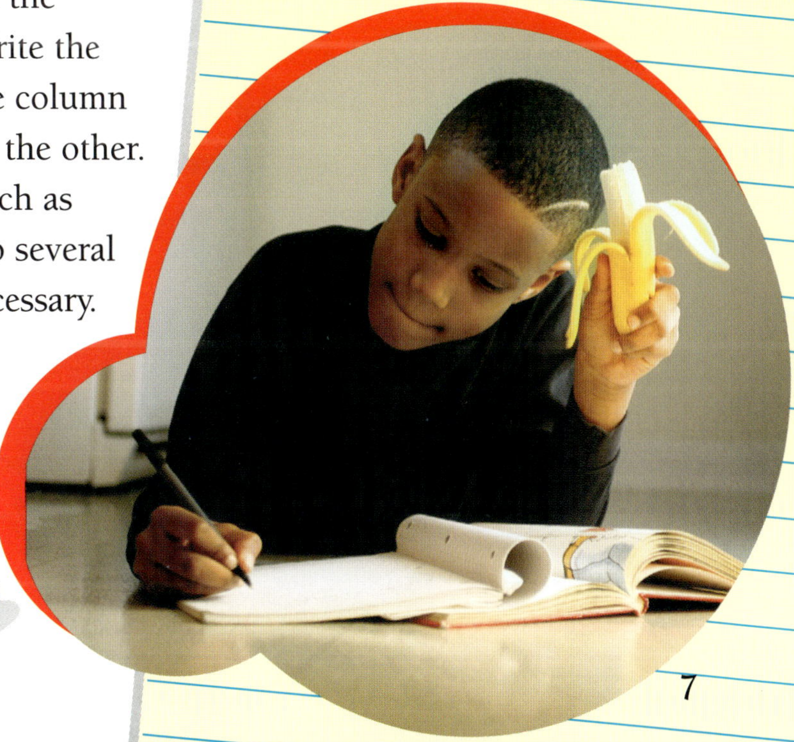

CHAPTER 1

A Balanced Diet

Because different foods have different kinds and amounts of nutrients, you need to eat a variety of foods every day to have a balanced diet. An apple is a healthful snack and a good source of some vitamins and minerals. But if you ate nothing but apples, you'd be missing other important nutrients.

How can you tell how much of different kinds of foods you should eat? The United States Department of Agriculture (USDA) developed a **food guide pyramid** that puts foods into six major groups and tells how much of each group is needed each day to stay healthy.

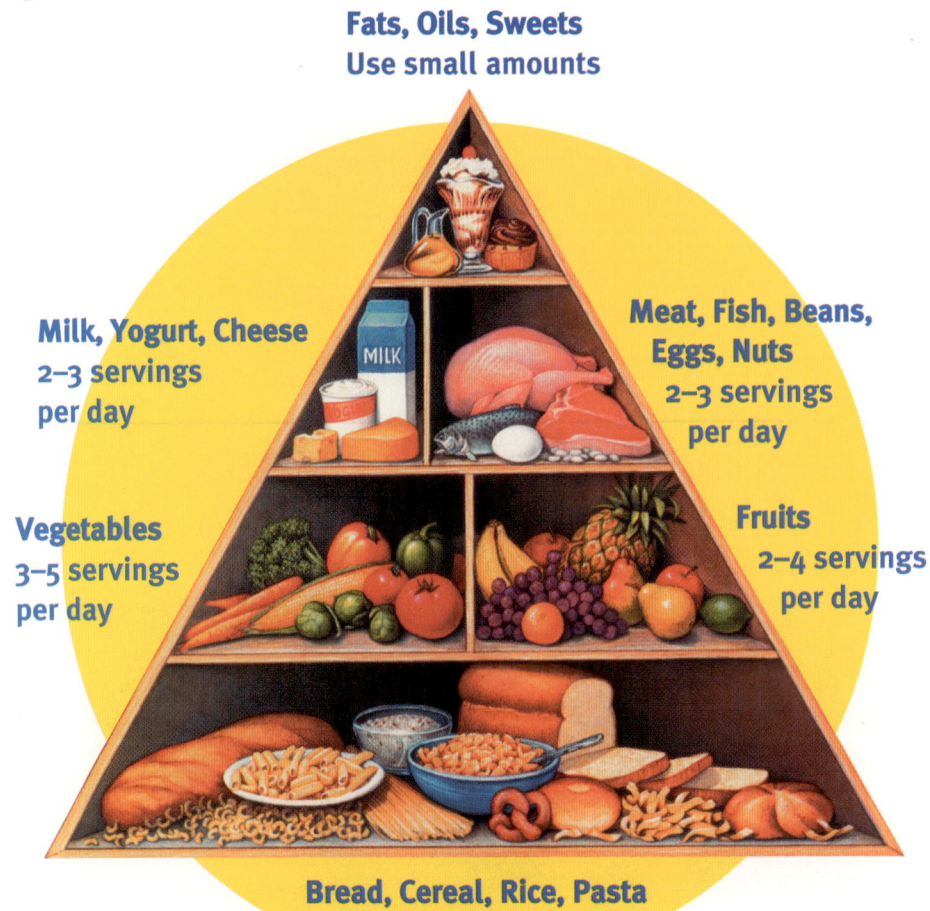

Fats, Oils, Sweets
Use small amounts

Milk, Yogurt, Cheese
2–3 servings per day

Meat, Fish, Beans, Eggs, Nuts
2–3 servings per day

Vegetables
3–5 servings per day

Fruits
2–4 servings per day

Bread, Cereal, Rice, Pasta
6–11 servings per day

FOOD FOR LIFE

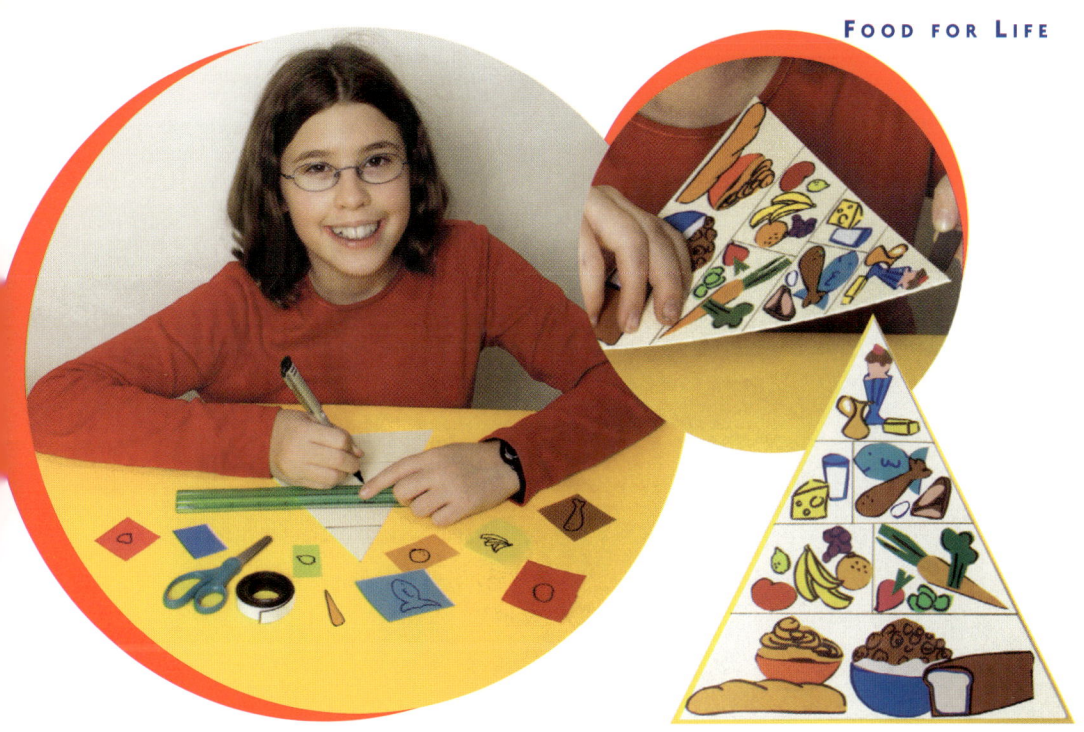

You should try to eat a balanced diet every day. To do this, you need to remember serving information.

Make a refrigerator magnet of the food guide pyramid.

What you need
- **poster board**
- **ruler**
- **scissors**
- **markers or crayons**
- **glue**
- **three flat magnets**

What to do

1. Cut a triangle with each side 8 inches long out of a piece of poster board.

2. To copy the food guide pyramid, make a horizontal line across the triangle every two inches. Draw a vertical line down the middle of the second and third sections of the triangle.

3. Copy the serving information from the food guide pyramid onto your model. Decorate each section with drawings of foods.

4. Glue three magnets to the back of the pyramid. Stick the magnet on your refrigerator to remind you how to eat a balanced diet!

CHAPTER 1

Wise Choices

Most foods contain more than one nutrient. How can you tell what nutrients are in a certain food? In 1990, a new law required packaged foods to have a label of nutrition facts. The label makes it easier for consumers to know exactly what they are eating.

Food labels list the nutrients in the food, as well as the ingredients. This helps you make wise choices about the foods you eat. You can compare foods and determine which one is more healthful. If you have special diet needs, a food label can help you choose or avoid foods.

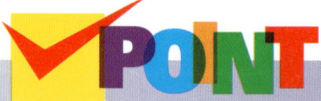

Think It Over

Compare these two snack food labels. Guess which one is for potato chips and which is for pretzels. Which food has a larger serving size? Which has more calories and fat per serving? Which vitamins are in each snack? Which is the healthier choice for a snack? NOTE: Be sure you are comparing the same size servings!

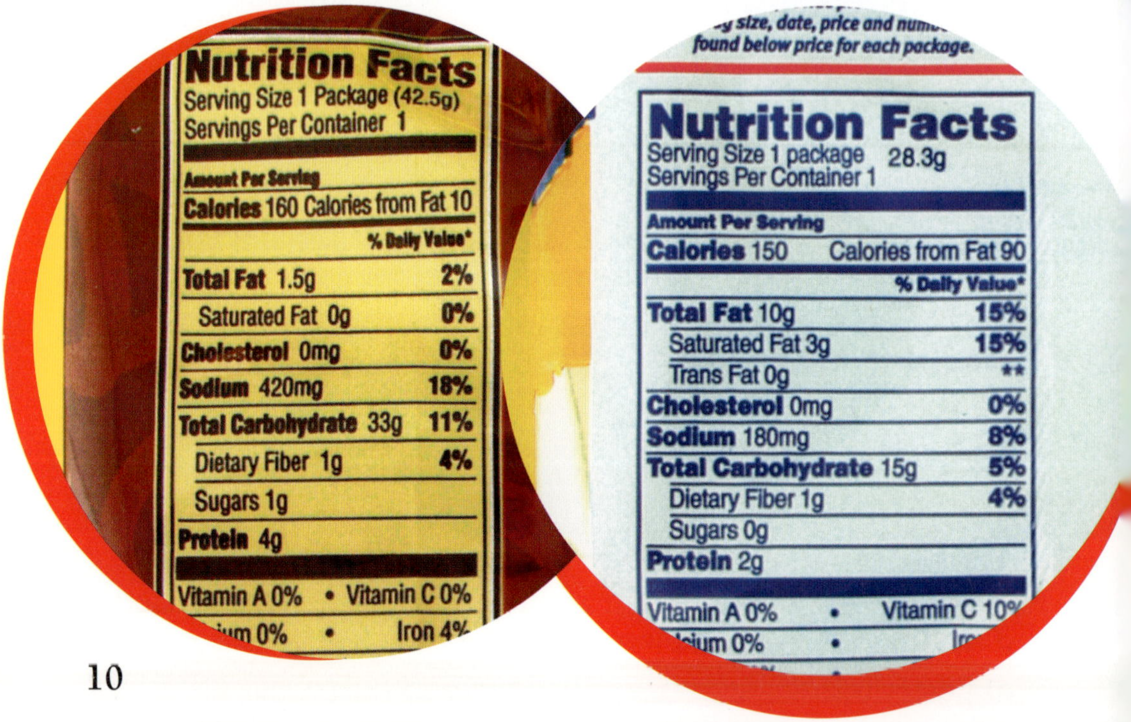

FOOD FOR LIFE

Try this activity to make healthful frozen orange-banana pops!

What you need
- **ice cube tray**
- **knife**
- **banana**
- **orange juice**
- **ice-cream pop stick**
- **freezer**

What to do

1. Ask an adult to cut a slice of banana for each section of the ice cube tray. Insert an ice-cream pop stick in each slice.

2. Place a stick-and-banana slice in each section of the ice cube tray. Then fill each section with orange juice.

3. Place the tray in the freezer. After 4 hours, remove the tray. To remove the banana-orange pops, bend each section of the tray.

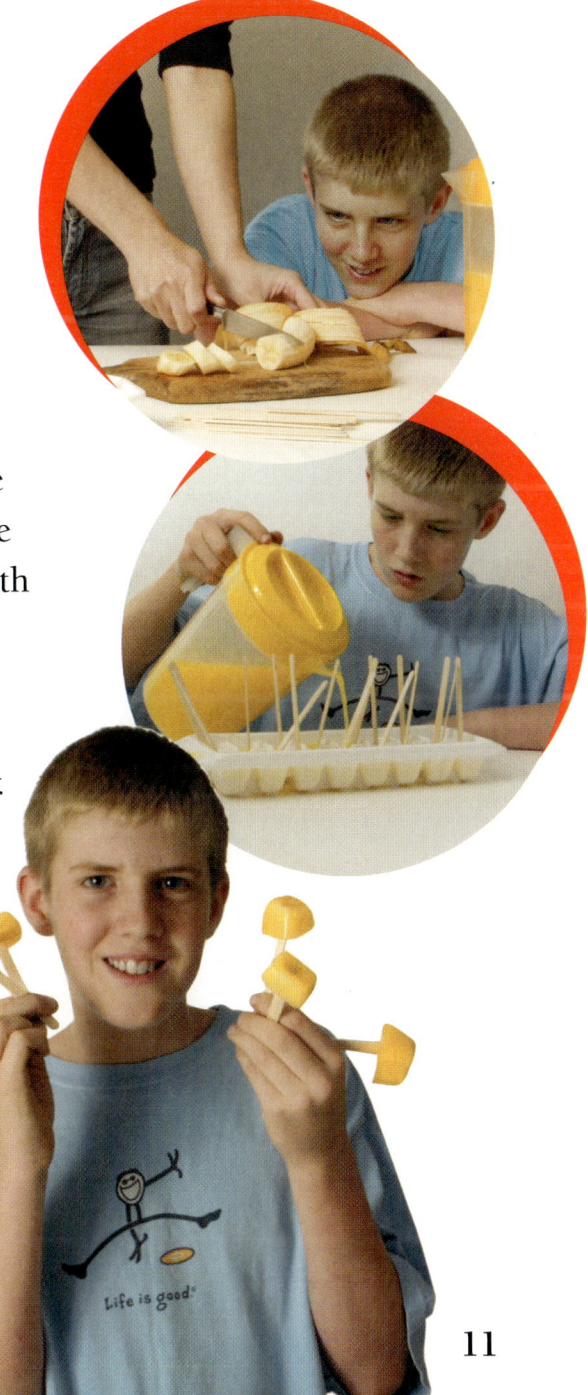

11

CHAPTER 2

Fitness for Life

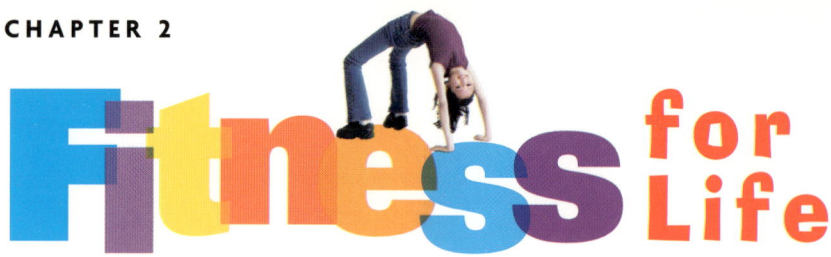

Developing good nutrition habits is only one way to stay healthy. Fitness is another important way to keep your body and mind in top form. Being fit keeps your body strong and flexible without letting it tire easily.

You can develop basic skills that will help you become fit in a safe and healthy way. Each skill involves your brain and body working together to do a task.

Skills such as **agility** and balance are needed if you want to skateboard and ski. **Coordination** and reaction time are used to get a hit in baseball. Speed and power are needed to win a relay race.

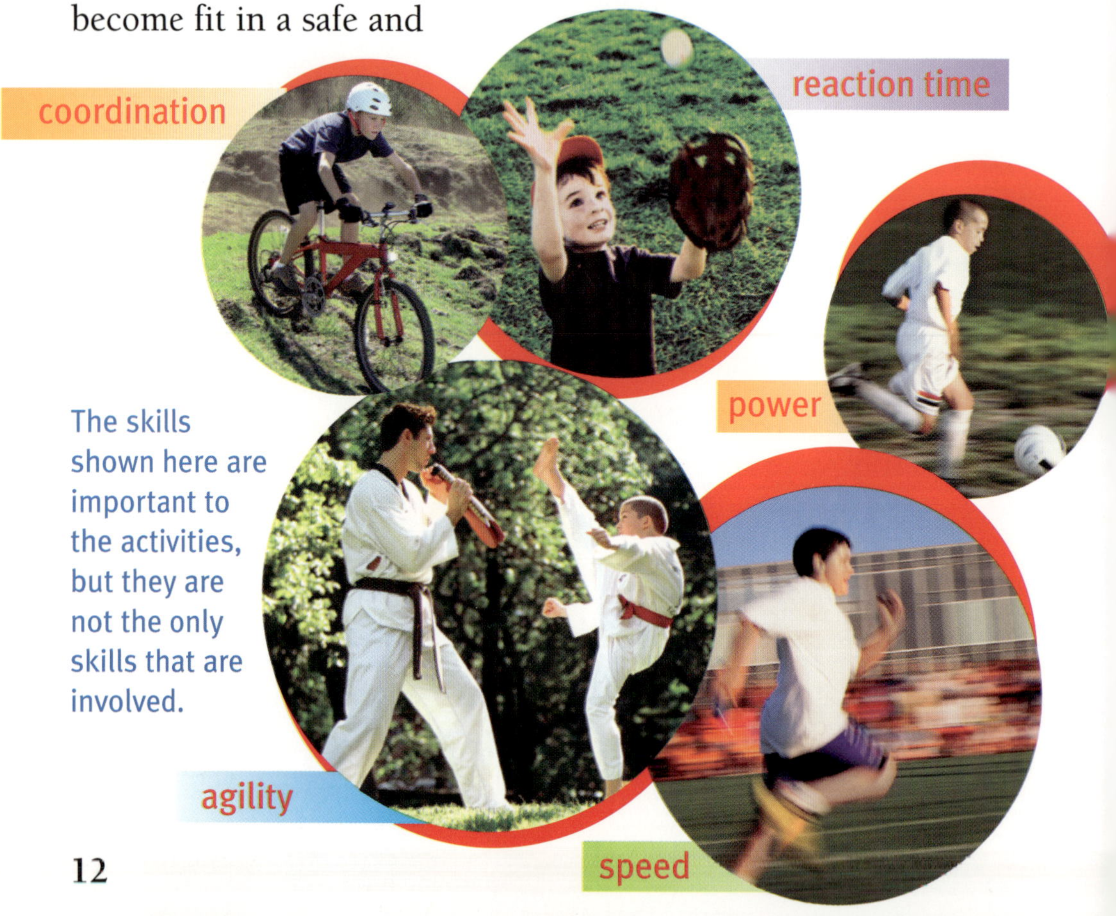

coordination

reaction time

power

The skills shown here are important to the activities, but they are not the only skills that are involved.

agility

speed

12

Try this experiment to test and practice reaction time.

What you need
- **thin cardboard**
- **ruler**
- **crayons**
- **scissors**

What to do

1. Cut a piece of thin cardboard into a 3-inch x 6-inch strip. Divide the strip into three sections of 2 inches each. From left to right, color the first section green, the second section red, and the third section blue.
2. Hold the strip vertically with the green section at the top. Have a partner hold his or her hand about three inches below the strip.
3. Drop the strip while your partner tries to grasp it before it hits the floor. Which colored section did your partner catch? Try it a few times and keep a record.
4. Switch places and try again. Use the scoring table below to see how you did.

 None = Try again!

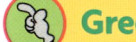 **Green = Good reaction time.**

 Red = Very good reaction time.

 Blue = Excellent reaction time!

CHAPTER 2

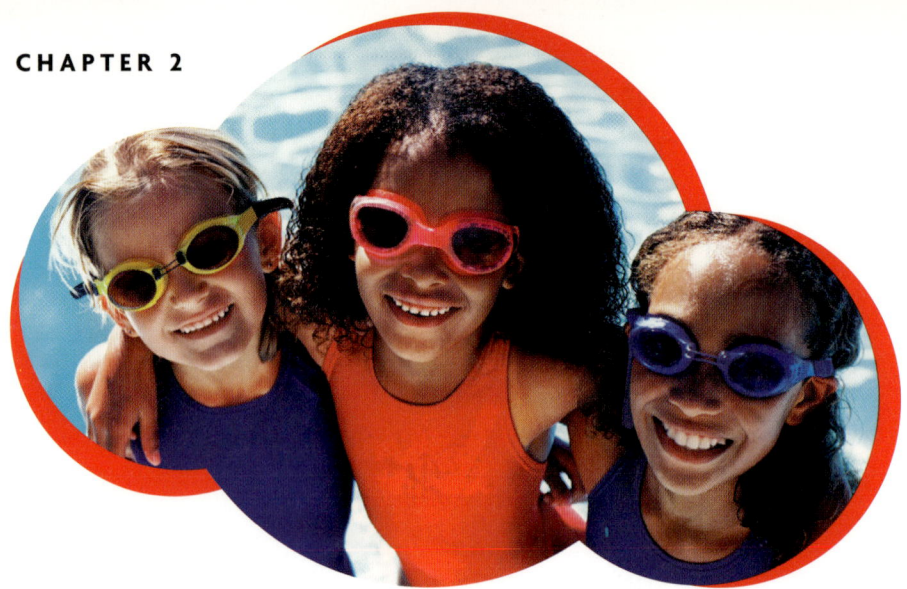

Getting Fit

Exercise is one way to become fit. There are several types of exercise. By increasing the rate at which your heart beats, **aerobic** exercise increases your endurance and strengthens your heart. It also improves your rate of breathing and can help lower your percentage of body fat.

During aerobic exercise, your body needs extra oxygen. To get the extra oxygen, you breathe faster. Running, walking, or biking at a steady pace for 20 minutes or more is aerobic exercise.

Anaerobic exercise helps develop speed and strength. Sprinting, downhill skiing, weight lifting, and baseball are anaerobic exercises. Your heart rate does not need to increase as much with this type of exercise.

What areas of fitness would you like to improve: strength, endurance, or both?

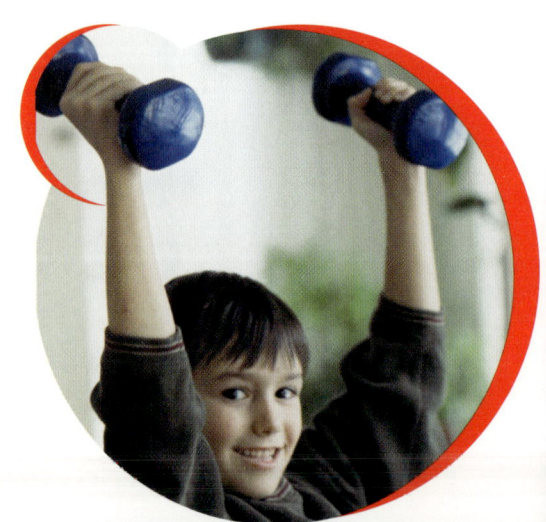

Try this activity to make a fitness diary to track your progress.

What you need
- **sheet of paper, 8½ inches x 11 inches**
- **pencil or pen**
- **markers**

What to do

1. Decide on the area of fitness you would like to improve.
2. To make the fitness diary, fold the sheet of paper in half lengthwise. Keeping it folded, turn each loose edge up toward the middle fold.
3. Now hold the paper lengthwise like a book. The outside column of paper is your diary cover. Decorate it as you wish.
4. Open the cover and label the top of each column with a day of the week. You have enough columns to keep track of your progress for five days.
5. At the end of the time, summarize what you did. Did you reach your goal? How can you improve the next time?

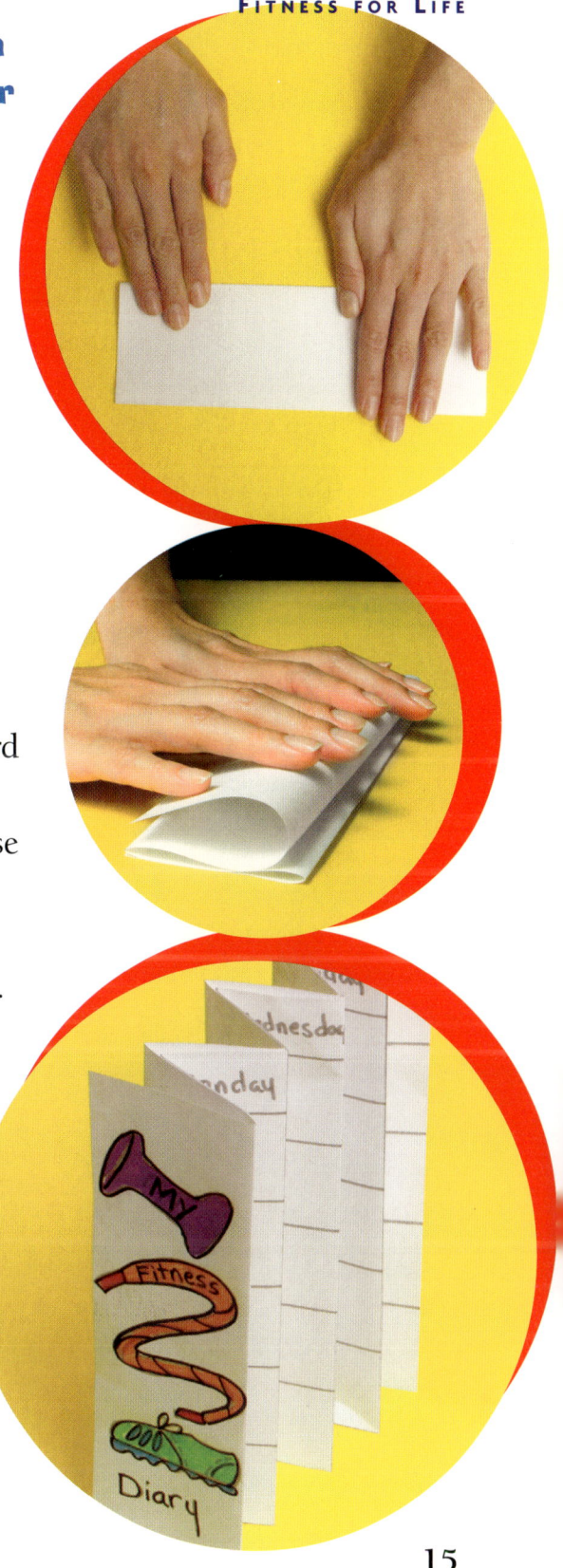

FITNESS FOR LIFE

15

CHAPTER 2

Exercising Safely

Helmets, shin guards, knee pads, and other safety equipment help protect your body and prevent injuries while you exercise. But this equipment must be used properly if it is to keep you safe.

To help avoid injuries while exercising, stretch and warm up your muscles first. Stretch your muscles slowly and carefully. You should not feel pain or strain.

Your heart is a muscle, too. Slowly increase your heart rate for three to five minutes before aerobic exercise. Walking or jogging slowly will increase your heart rate. After your workout, take three to five minutes to cool down. This allows your heart rate to return to normal.

Your **pulse** shows the rate at which your heart is beating. You can feel your pulse by gently placing two fingers at the side of your neck or on the underside of your wrist.

IT'S A FACT!

You need to replace your water supply! Your body loses about 10 cups of water a day, and more when you exercise. Drink a glass of water before exercising. Drink more every 20 minutes or if you're tired or thirsty.

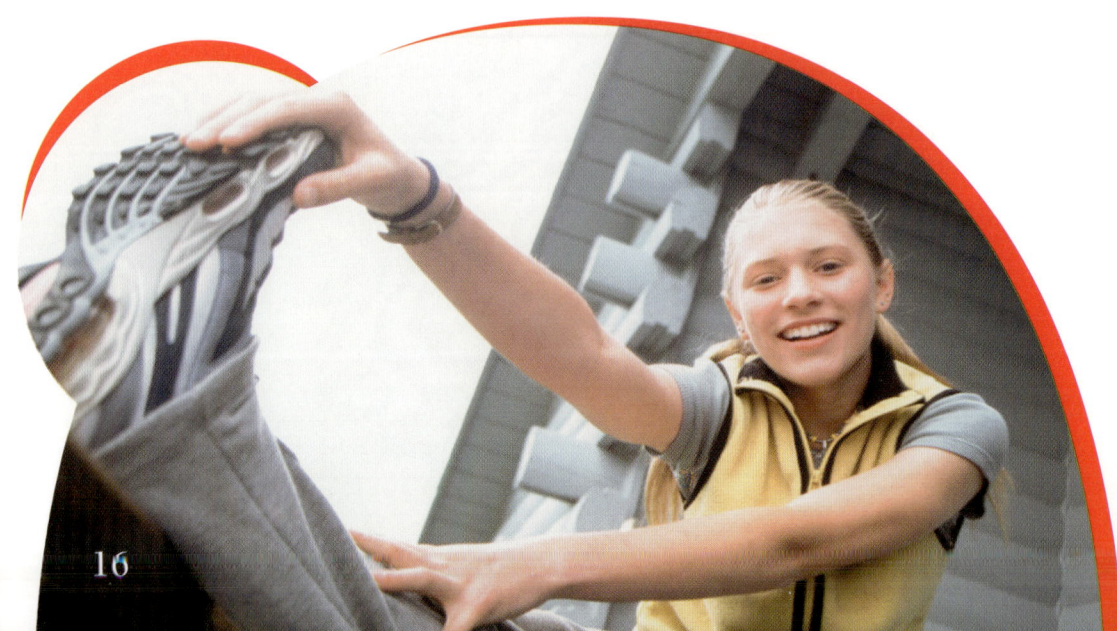

FITNESS FOR LIFE

Try this activity to find out how your heart rate changes before, during, and after exercise.

What you need
- **sneakers**
- **stop watch**
- **pencil**
- **paper**

What to do

1. Find your pulse by placing your index and middle fingers on the underside of your wrist.
2. Record the number of pulses, or beats, you feel in 15 seconds while resting. You might want to do this two or three times to make sure you are counting correctly. Multiply this number by four to find the number of times your heart beats in one minute.
3. Run in place for one minute. As soon as you stop, repeat step 2.
4. Wait one more minute. Repeat step 2.
5. Repeat step 4 several times until your heart rate has returned to your starting rate. Make a line graph to record your results.

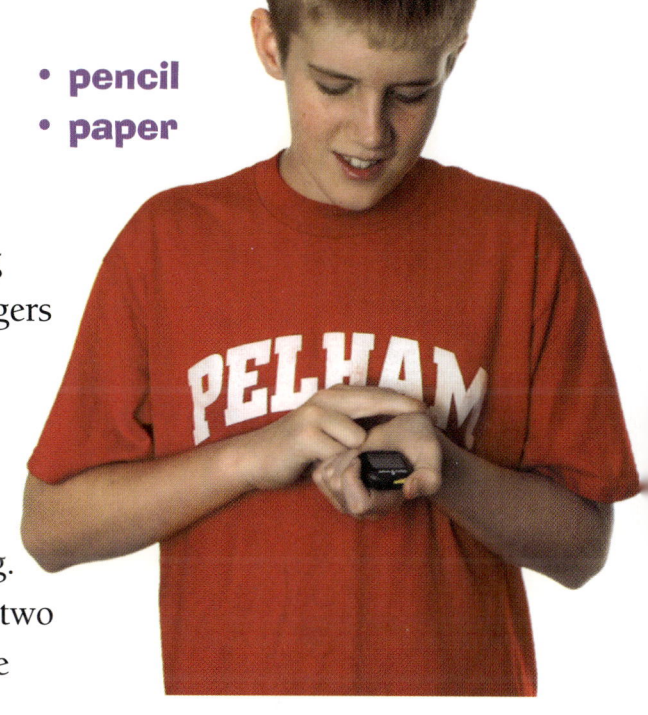

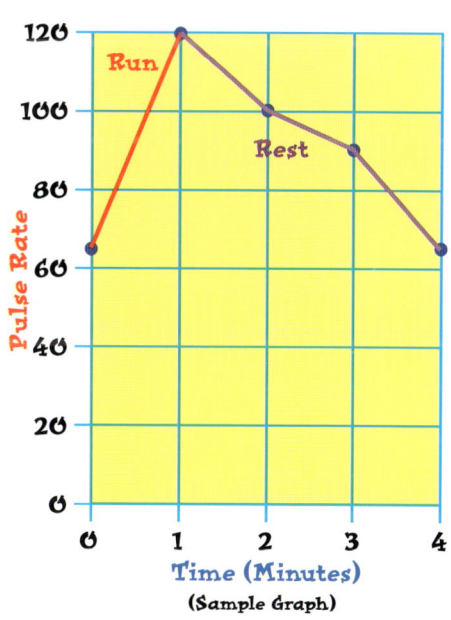

(Sample Graph)

CHAPTER 3

A Healthy Look

Most healthy people look healthy. There are many habits you can practice that will give you a healthy look.

One important habit is to use sunscreen on your skin when you go out in the sun. Another is to get enough sleep and rest so that you are not tired. Have checkups with your doctor, dentist, and eye doctor regularly.

Keeping neat and clean is part of grooming. Here are some things you can do to practice good grooming.

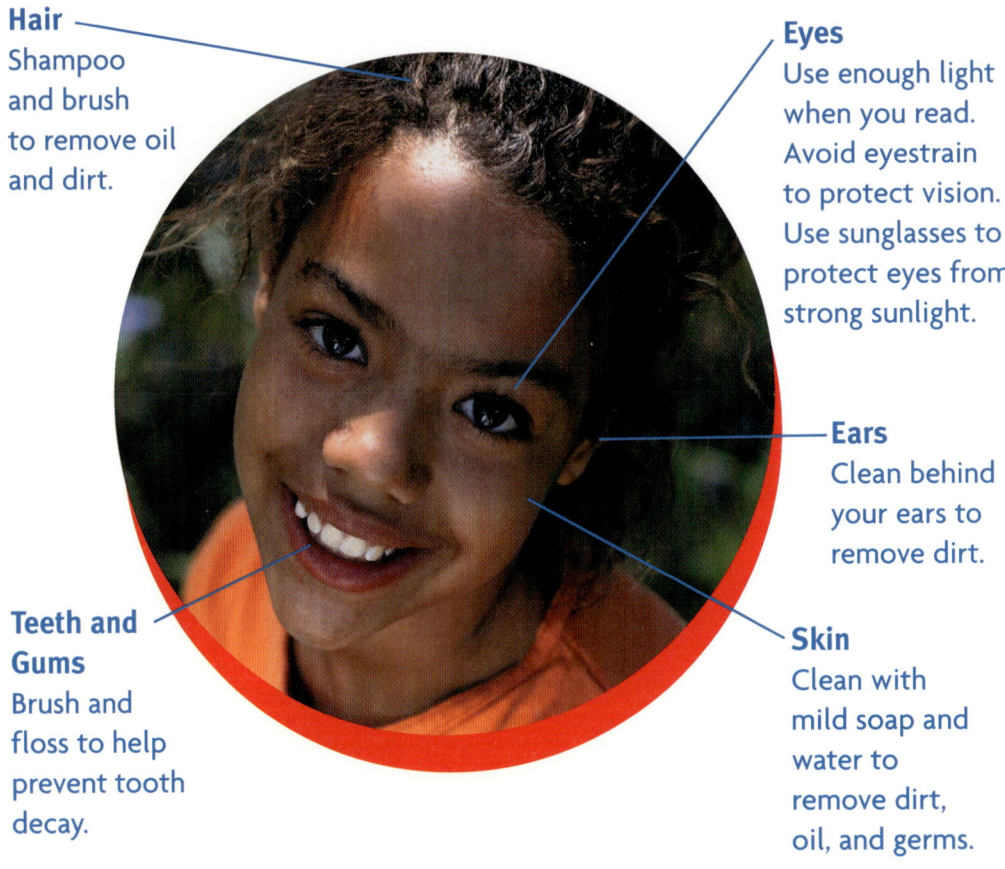

Hair
Shampoo and brush to remove oil and dirt.

Teeth and Gums
Brush and floss to help prevent tooth decay.

Eyes
Use enough light when you read. Avoid eyestrain to protect vision. Use sunglasses to protect eyes from strong sunlight.

Ears
Clean behind your ears to remove dirt.

Skin
Clean with mild soap and water to remove dirt, oil, and germs.

When you brush your teeth, most pieces of food are removed with your toothbrush. But some pieces can get caught between the teeth. Germs can act on this trapped food and form **plaque**. Flossing helps get rid of plaque and removes food that can cause cavities.

IT'S A FACT!

Your eyes and ears are self-cleaning. Never put anything in your eyes or ears. Have your ears checked and see an eye doctor once a year.

Try this activity to make sure you are flossing correctly.

What you need
- **dental floss**
- **mirror**

What to do

1. Use a piece of floss about 12 inches long. Wind each end gently around the middle finger of each hand.
2. Hold the floss tightly between your fingers. Place the floss between two teeth.
3. Use a gentle motion to move the floss up and down between the teeth. Wrap the floss slightly around one tooth and move it toward your gum line.
4. Repeat steps 2 and 3 for each tooth. Ask an adult for help if you are having trouble or if the flossing hurts.

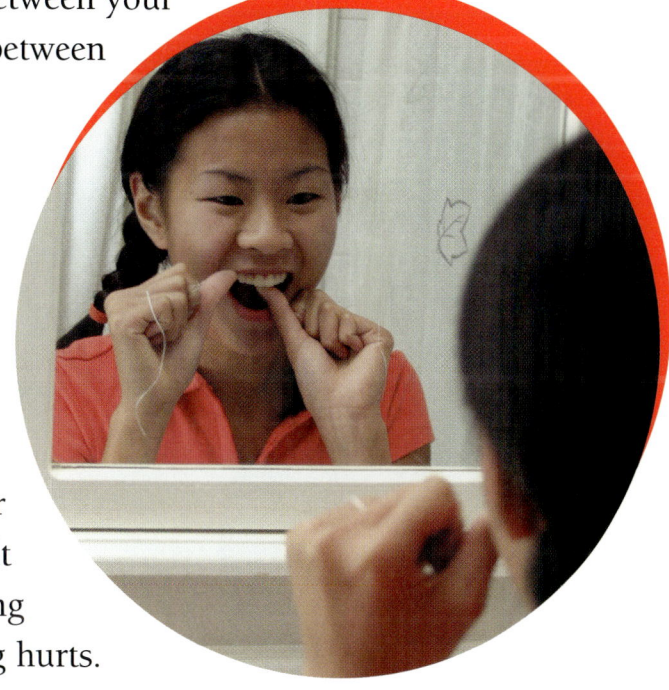

CHAPTER 3

Good posture contributes to a healthy look and has health benefits, too. Correct posture can help prevent backaches. It also gives your internal organs room to work properly. It allows blood to flow to your organs easily.

Practice good posture by standing with your neck, shoulders, lower back, and hips in line with one another.

Taking care of your nails is also part of good grooming. Make sure your fingernails and toenails are clean. Keep dirt from getting under the nails when you are working with messy materials or walking barefoot. Keeping your nails clean can help prevent nail infections. Keep nails trimmed or filed so they do not easily break or tear.

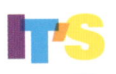

Fingernails grow at an average rate of 3 millimeters per month. It takes six months for a fingernail to completely regrow. Toenails take two to three times longer to grow because blood does not flow to them as well.

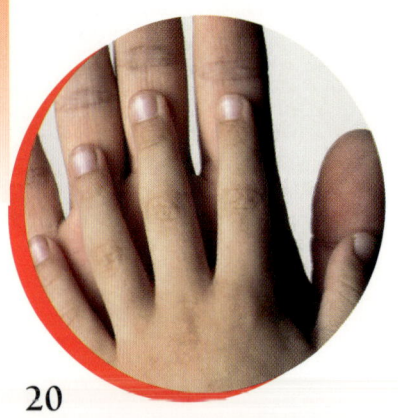

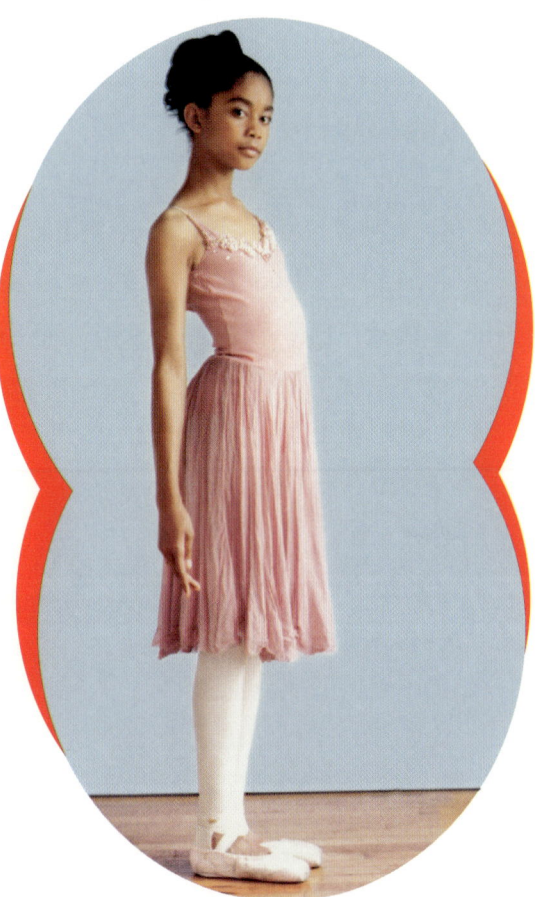

Good posture is beneficial to good health.

CHAPTER 4

Preventing Illness

Some people are born with diseases they will have their whole lives. Many others develop diseases later in life. These diseases include cancer, diabetes, heart disease, and arthritis. Such diseases are called **noncommunicable**. They cannot be spread from person to person.

Other diseases are called **communicable** diseases because they can be spread from person to person. They are caused by germs. Germs are **microscopic**, too small to be seen with the unaided eye. Most germs are harmless, but some can make you sick.

Bacteria	Strep throat, ear infection
Virus	Colds, flu, measles
Protozoa	Malaria
Fungus	Athlete's foot, nail infections, ringworm

This chart lists some diseases and the organisms that cause them.

These are bacteria magnified thousands of times.

21

CHAPTER 4

Communicable diseases can be spread in several ways. Some germs travel through the air or on objects. Some are spread in food, water, and living things.

Your body has its own natural ways of fighting disease. But if you develop helpful habits for disease prevention, you can often avoid exposure to harmful germs.

The best thing you can do is keep away from germs. That means staying away from people who are sick with communicable diseases that are easily transmitted.

It also means not sharing food, silverware, or cups and glasses with other people. Washing your hands with soap and water before eating is another good habit to practice. You should always wash your hands with soap and water when you are around someone who is sick. If you are sick, you should wash your hands often.

IT'S A FACT!

Some diseases, such as polio, are very rare in the United States because of **vaccines**. Many vaccines, which are usually given in the form of an injection, contain a very weak or killed form of a disease-causing organism. The vaccine prevents you from getting the particular disease for a period of time.

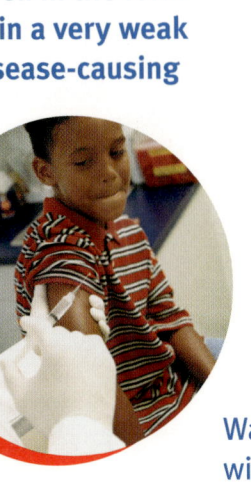

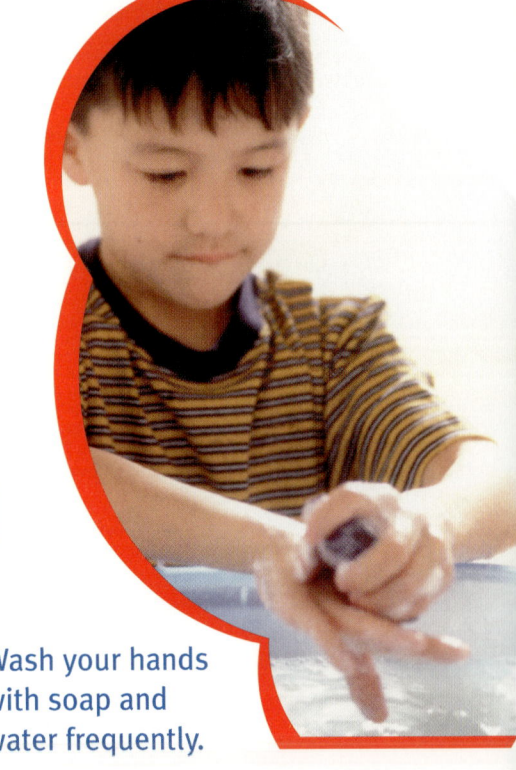

Wash your hands with soap and water frequently.

22

PREVENTING ILLNESS

This activity will show you the difference between washing with soap and water and washing with water alone.

What you need
- **petroleum jelly or moisturizer**
- **dish of sand**

What to do
1. Coat your hands with a thin layer of petroleum jelly or moisturizer.
2. Press one hand into a dish of sand and gently rub your hands together. The sand represents germs on your skin.
3. Predict what might happen if you attempt to wash off the sand using only water. Try it.
4. Predict what might happen if you use soap and water to wash off the sand. Try it. Report your results.

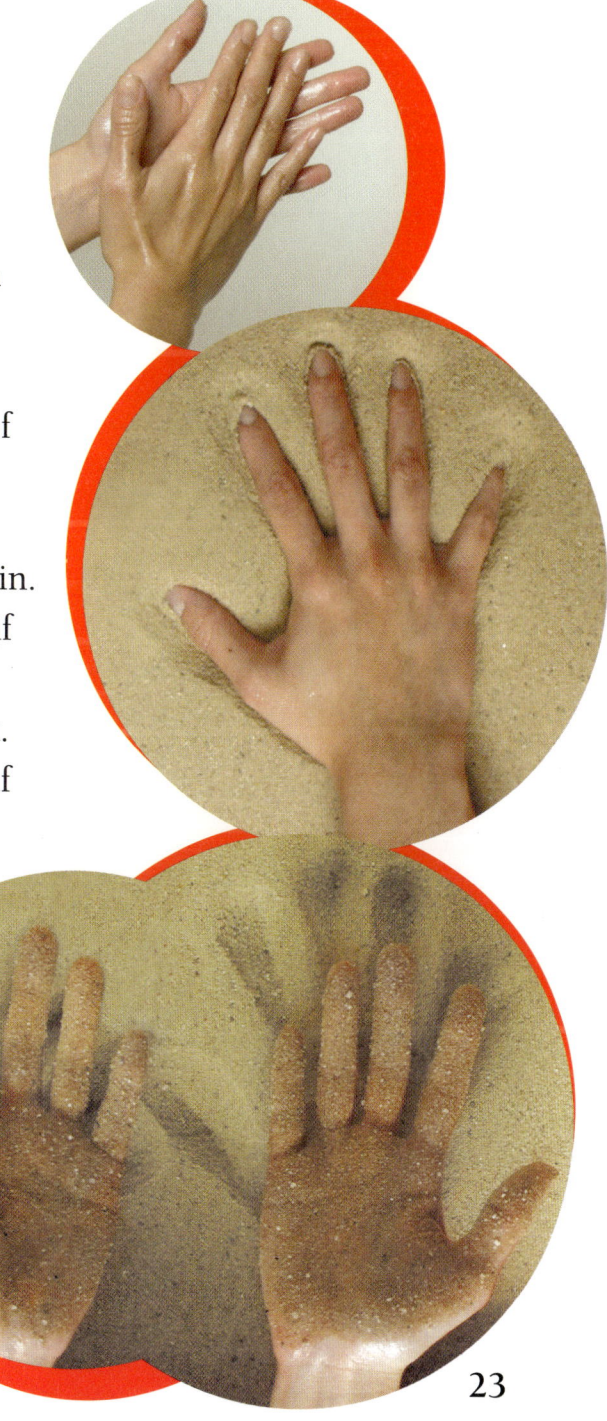

23

CHAPTER 5

Safety and First Aid

Why do you think it is important to follow rules about safety? You are correct if you said to avoid injury. Many injuries occur because people don't know how to stay safe.

Suppose your friend asks you to go biking in an area you know is dangerous, near a construction site or on a road that has lots of traffic perhaps. What should you say? If you are aware of the possible dangers to you and your friend, you will avoid such situations. In that way, you will be staying safe.

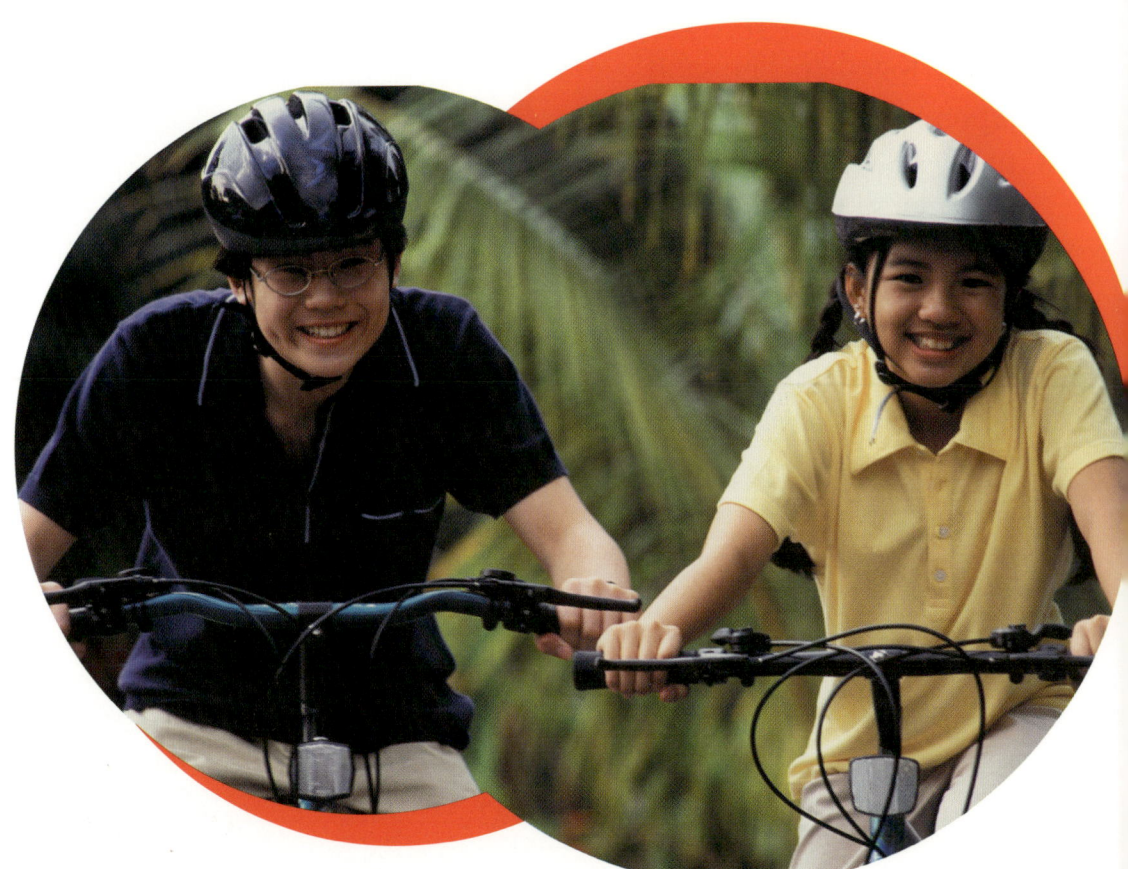

STAYING SAFE

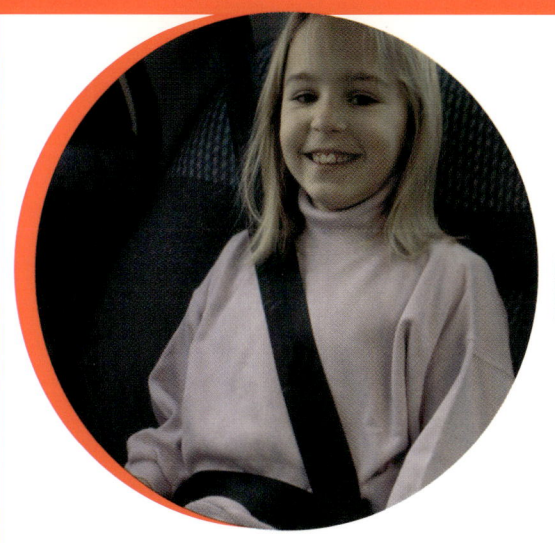
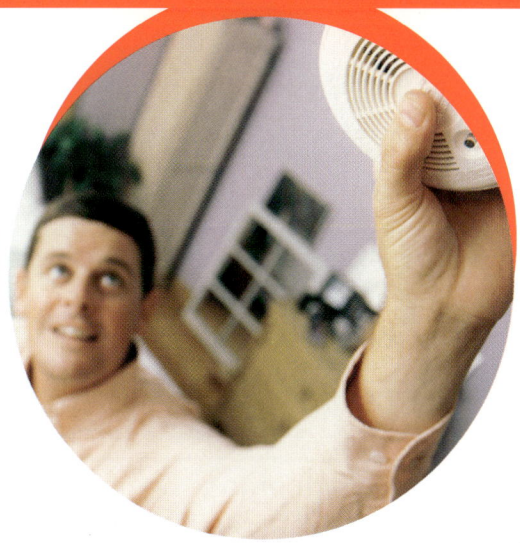

Car Safety
Always wear your seat belt. Don't distract the driver. Sit in the back seat. More than 4 million emergency-room visits each year are due to car accidents.

Fire Safety
Make sure smoke detectors have working batteries. Find fire escape routes from several places in your home. Do not cook or work in the kitchen without help from an adult.

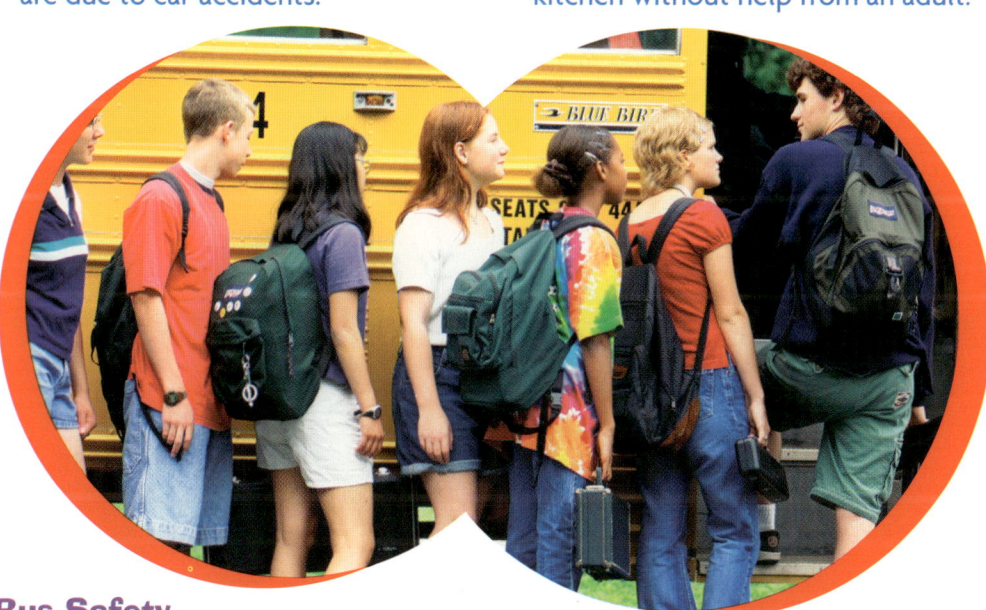

Bus Safety
Wait for the bus to come to a complete stop before going near it. Stay seated while the bus is moving. Keep your arms inside the window at all times. Cross the street at least 10 feet in front of the stopped bus. Look for cars and traffic before crossing. Most school-bus injuries happen when students are getting on or off the bus.

CHAPTER 5

One important part of staying safe is making sure that people around you follow safety rules, too.

Try this activity to inform other students of safety rules.

What you need
- **poster board**
- **crayons**
- **research materials**

What to do

1. In a small group, review the pictures on the opposite page. Choose one situation for which you will make an informative safety poster to display at school.

2. Brainstorm ideas about how to stay safe in that situation. Use research materials or the Internet to find other rules you may not know about.

3. Illustrate the poster and write the safety rules underneath it. Be sure to use language that can be understood by students younger than you. Give the poster a title.

4. Hang your poster and those of your classmates in the hallway at school.

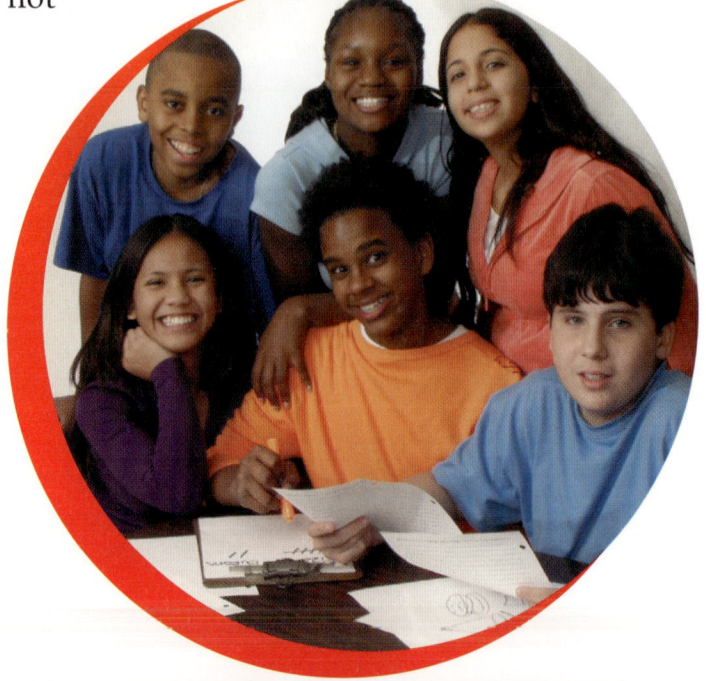

SAFETY AND FIRST AID

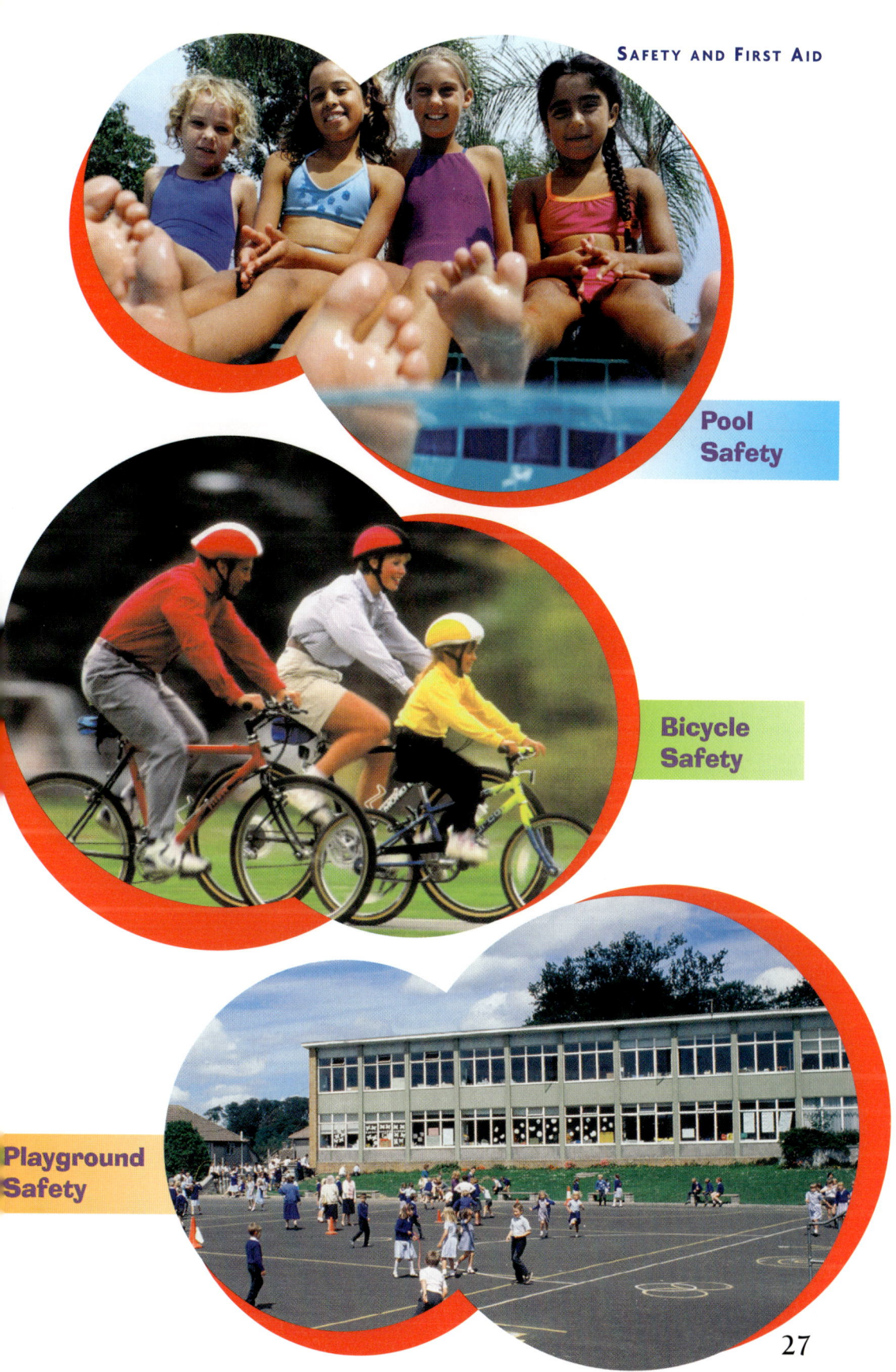

Pool Safety

Bicycle Safety

Playground Safety

27

CHAPTER 5

When an injury occurs, there are some actions you can take right away. Most minor cuts, scrapes, bruises, nosebleeds, insect bites, and stings are injuries that can be treated with first aid. Some insect stings and other injuries require help from a doctor or other adult.

Following the rules shown here will allow you to give first aid to yourself or an injured person.

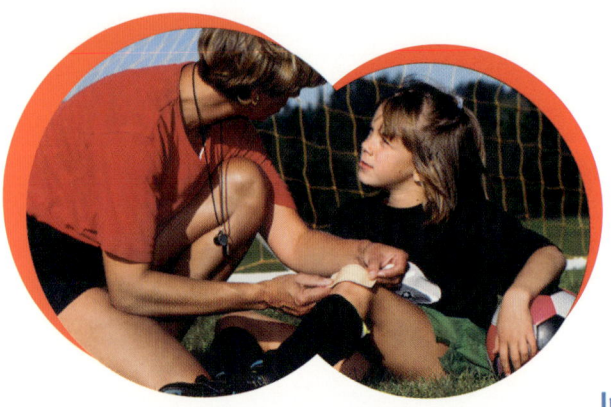

Cuts Clean the cut with soap and water. Apply a clean cloth or bandage and light pressure. See a doctor if the cut does not stop bleeding soon.

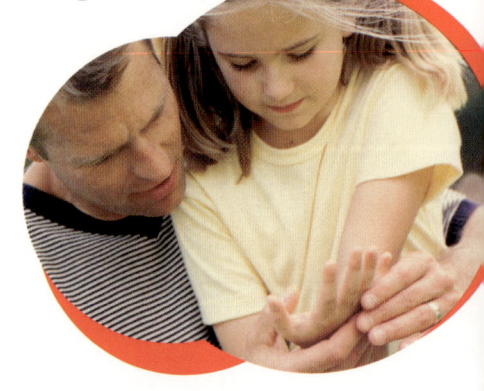

Insect bites and stings Apply an ice pack to the area. See a doctor if the swelling does not go down. For some people, insect stings are life-threatening. Immediate medical attention is necessary.

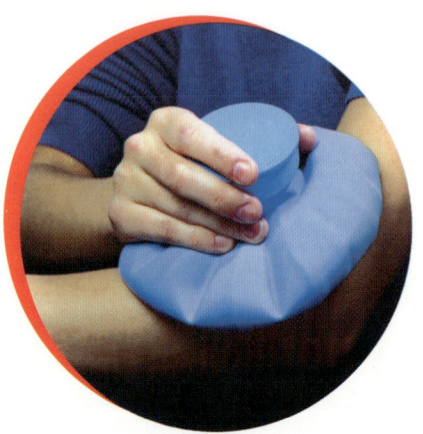

Bruises Apply a cold cloth or ice pack to the area. See a doctor if you have trouble moving the bruised area.

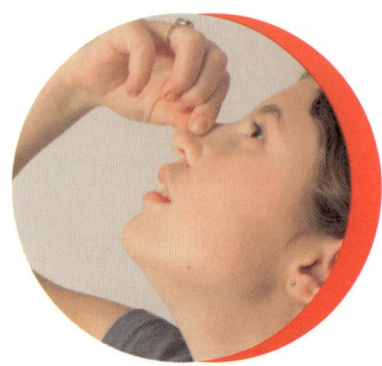

Nosebleeds Keep your head back. Apply light pressure to the bridge of your nose. See a doctor if the nosebleed does not stop.

SAFETY AND FIRST AID

In order for a person to give first aid, the right supplies are needed.

Make your own first-aid kit.

What you need
- box
- craft materials
- gauze
- first-aid solution
- bandages
- scissors
- clean cloth

What to do
1. Choose a box for a first-aid kit. Make sure it closes tightly so that the items inside stay clean. Decorate the box if you wish, using craft materials and pictures.
2. Collect supplies for your kit. These can include adhesive bandages, gauze, clean cloth, and first-aid solution.
3. Decide on the best place to keep your kit. It could go in the kitchen, the family car, the classroom, or other places.
4. Let people know where you have put your first-aid kit. Have them check it and make suggestions about items they think should be included. They may need to use your kit someday.

IT'S A FACT!

Most areas of the United States have a number that can be called in emergency situations. That number is 911 and it can be dialed free-of-charge. If you have to use the emergency number, remember the following:
- stay calm
- speak slowly and clearly
- follow the directions of the operator

If you live in an area without 911 service, you can dial zero and the operator will help. Remember, 911 is for real emergencies only!

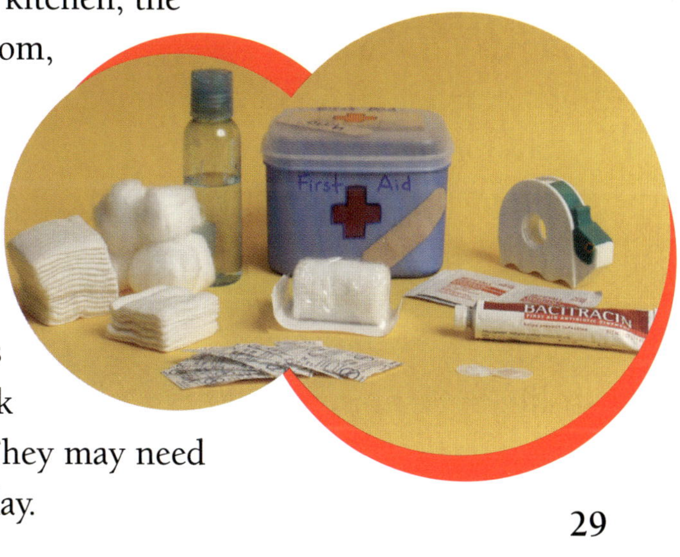

CONCLUSION

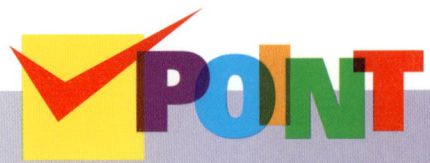

Make Connections

Create a *Healthy Me* book to show what you have learned about staying healthy.

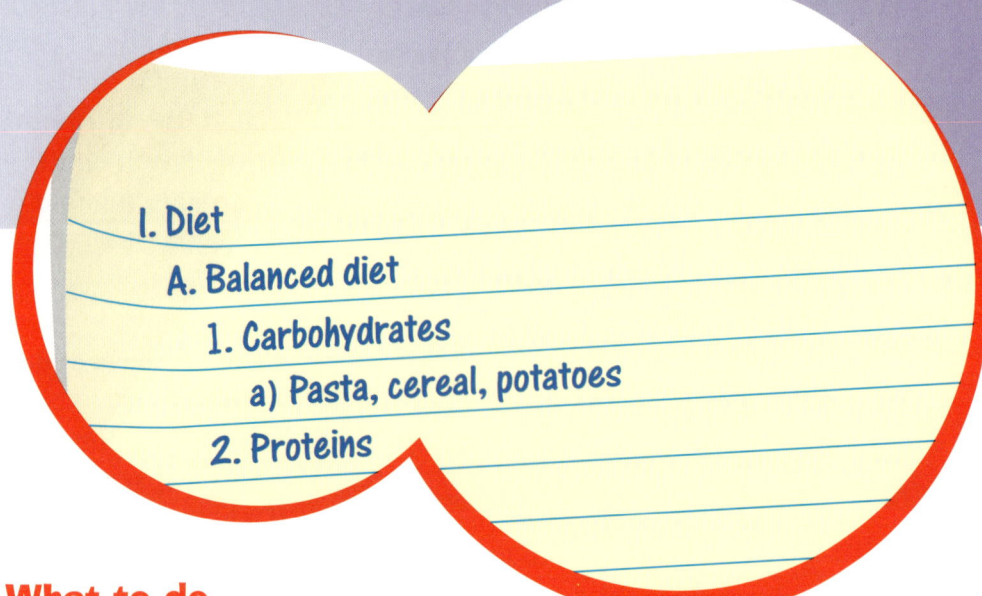

What to do

1. Outline the topics you would like to cover in your book. Include something for each chapter that you read: diet, fitness, grooming, disease prevention, and safety and first aid. Decide how many pages you will need for each topic.
2. Write about each topic and include illustrations or pictures cut from old magazines. Use graphs or charts to explain information visually.
3. Include a chapter on a health topic that was not discussed in this book. Research the topic and write about it in your book.
4. Gather the finished pages and staple them together. Design and attach a colorful construction-paper cover.

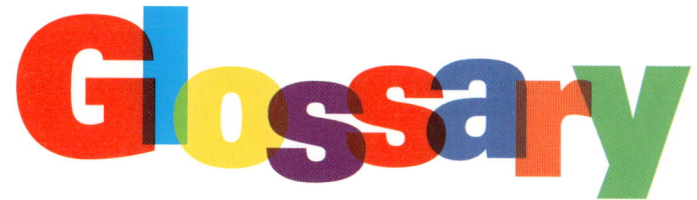

aerobic	(uh-ROH-bihk) an activity or exercise that increases heart and breathing rates (page 14)
agility	(uh-JIL-i-tee) the ability to move easily and quickly (page 12)
anaerobic	(ANN-uh-roh-bihk) an activity or exercise that does not involve increased breathing or oxygen (page 14)
communicable	(KUH-mue-nih-kuh-bul) able to be spread from person to person (page 21)
coordination	(KO-or-di-nay-shun) the ability of parts to work well together (page 12)
food guide pyramid	(FOOD GIGHD PIHR-uh-mid) a guide to healthful eating provided by the United States Department of Agriculture (page 8)
microscopic	(MY-crow-SCOP-ihk) able to be seen only through a microscope (page 21)
noncommunicable	(NON-kuh-mue-nih-kuh-bul) unable to be spread from person to person (page 21)
nutrient	(NOO-tree-ehnt) a substance in foods used by the body (page 6)
plaque	(PLAK) a sticky material that forms on teeth (page 19)
pulse	(PUHLS) the regular, rhythmic beating of the heart that can be felt at certain points on the body (page 16)
vaccine	(VAK-seen) a medication of a killed, or weakened germ that decreases the likelihood of the disease in that organism (page 22)
wellness	(WELL-nehs) the state of being in good health (page 2)

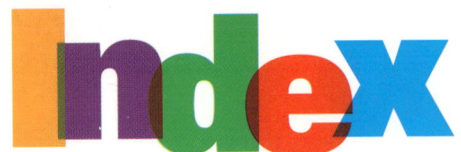

aerobic, 14, 16

agility, 12

anaerobic, 14

carbohydrate, 6–7

communicable, 21–22

coordination, 12

disease, 21–23

emotions, 2–3

fats, 6–7, 8, 14

first aid, 24, 28–29

fitness, 4–5, 12, 14–16

floss, 19

food guide pyramid, 8–9

food label, 10

germs, 18, 19, 21–23

grooming, 4–5, 18, 20, 30

habits, 4, 12, 18, 22

heart rate, 14, 16–17

illness prevention, 4, 22–23

mental health, 2–3

microscopic, 21

minerals, 6–7, 8

noncommunicable, 21

nutrients, 6–7, 8, 10

nutrition, 4–5, 12

physical health, 2, 4–5

plaque, 19

posture, 20

proteins, 6–7

pulse, 16–17

safety, 4–5, 16, 24–28

serving size, 8, 10

social health, 2–3

stress, 3

USDA, 8

vaccine, 22

vitamins, 6–7, 8

water, 6–7, 16, 22

wellness, 2